Weight Loss Guide

The definitive guide to a
sustainable weight loss

Melissa Fogel

Table of Contents

Introduction

John had been struggling with his weight for years. No matter what diet and fitness plan he followed, nothing seemed to work. He was starting to feel hopeless.

One day, John was browsing the internet when he came across a weight loss guide. The guide was written by a doctor who had helped thousands of people lose weight. John was intrigued, so he decided to give it a try.

The guide was full of practical advice and tips. It covered everything from diet and exercise to stress management and motivation. John found the guide to be very helpful. He started following the advice in the guide, and he soon began to see results.

After a few months, John had lost a significant amount of weight. He was feeling healthier and more confident than he had in years. He was so grateful to the weight loss guide for helping him achieve his goals.

One day, John was walking down the street when he saw a woman he had known in high school. He hadn't seen her in years, but he recognized her immediately.

"Hey," John said. "It's me, John."

The woman looked at him for a moment, and then her eyes widened in surprise. "John!" she said. "You look amazing! What have you been doing?"

John smiled. "I've been following a weight loss guide," he said. "It's really helped me."

The woman smiled back. "Well, it's definitely working," she said. "You look great."

John thanked her, and they talked for a few minutes. As they parted ways, John felt a sense of satisfaction. He knew that he had made a big change in his life, and he was proud of himself for sticking with it.

John continued to follow the advice in the weight loss guide, and he eventually reached his goal weight. He was so happy with the results that he decided to share his story with others. He started a blog and wrote about his weight loss journey. He also started speaking at conferences and workshops.

John's story has inspired thousands of people to lose weight and improve their health. He is proof that it is possible to achieve your weight loss goals, no matter how difficult they may seem.

Losing weight can be a challenging journey, but it is an important one for many individuals. In this guide, we will explore the reasons why losing weight is important and the numerous benefits that come with achieving a healthy weight. We will also delve into the science behind weight loss, including the factors that affect it and how to set realistic goals. Understanding nutrition is crucial when it comes to weight loss, so we will discuss the role of diet in achieving your desired weight. We will provide a comprehensive list of foods that you should include in your weight loss diet, such as fruits and vegetables, whole grains and legumes, lean protein sources, healthy fats and oils, and low-calorie snacks and desserts. Additionally, we will highlight foods that you should limit or avoid, such as sugary and processed foods, high-fat and fried foods, alcohol, and sugary drinks.

Exercise and physical activity play a significant role in weight loss as well, so we will emphasize their importance and explore different types of exercises that can aid in shedding pounds. This includes cardiovascular exercises, strength training exercises, and flexibility and balance exercises. We will also guide you through creating a personalized exercise plan that suits your needs and preferences.

Behavior and lifestyle changes are essential for long-term weight loss success, so we will provide strategies for mindful eating, portion control, meal planning and preparation, overcoming emotional eating, managing stress, and improving sleep quality.

Tracking progress and staying motivated are key components of any weight loss journey. We will discuss how to monitor your weight loss progress, celebrate milestones and non-scale victories, overcome plateaus and setbacks, and find support and accountability.

Finally, we will delve into sustainable weight loss and maintenance strategies to help you create a long-term healthy lifestyle. We will provide tips for maintaining weight loss, navigating eating out and social situations, and offer resources and further information to support you on your journey.

By the end of this guide, you will have the knowledge and tools necessary to embark on a successful weight loss journey and achieve your desired goals. Let's get started!

Reasons Why Losing Weight is Important

Losing weight is important for several reasons, both for our physical and mental well-being. Here are some key reasons why achieving a healthy weight is crucial:

1. Improved overall health: Excess weight can increase the risk of developing various health conditions such as heart disease, type 2 diabetes, high blood pressure, certain types of cancer, and sleep apnea. By losing weight, you can reduce the risk of these diseases and improve your overall health.

2. Increased energy levels: Carrying excess weight can make you feel sluggish and fatigued. Losing weight can boost your energy levels, allowing

you to engage in physical activities with greater ease and enjoy a more active lifestyle.

3. Enhanced mood and mental well-being: Weight loss has been shown to improve mood and reduce symptoms of depression and anxiety. Achieving a healthy weight can boost self-confidence and improve body image, leading to improved mental well-being.

4. Better sleep quality: Obesity is often associated with sleep disorders such as sleep apnea and insomnia. Losing weight can alleviate these issues, leading to better sleep quality and overall restfulness.

5. Reduced joint pain: Carrying excess weight puts additional strain on your joints, leading to joint pain and increased risk of conditions like

osteoarthritis. Losing weight can relieve this strain, reducing joint pain and improving mobility.

6. Increased longevity: Studies have shown that maintaining a healthy weight can increase life expectancy. By reducing the risk of chronic diseases and improving overall health, weight loss can contribute to a longer and healthier life.

The Benefits of Achieving a Healthy Weight

Achieving a healthy weight comes with numerous benefits that can positively impact various aspects of your life. Here are some key benefits:

1. Improved physical fitness: Losing weight can improve your physical fitness by increasing strength, endurance, and flexibility. This allows you to engage in physical activities with greater ease and enjoy a more active lifestyle.

2. Enhanced self-confidence: Achieving a healthy weight can boost self-confidence and improve body image. Feeling good about your appearance can positively impact your overall self-esteem and quality of life.

3. Increased mobility: Carrying excess weight can make simple tasks like walking or climbing stairs challenging. Losing weight can improve mobility, making daily activities easier and more enjoyable.

4. Better heart health: Losing weight can reduce the risk of heart disease by lowering blood pressure, cholesterol levels, and the strain on the heart. This leads to improved cardiovascular health and a reduced risk of heart-related complications.

5. Improved digestion and gut health: A healthy weight is associated with improved digestion and a reduced risk of digestive disorders such as acid reflux, constipation, and irritable bowel syndrome (IBS).

6. Enhanced fertility: For individuals struggling with infertility, achieving a healthy weight can improve fertility by regulating hormone levels and increasing the chances of successful conception.

7.   Reduced   healthcare   costs: Maintaining a healthy weight can lead to reduced healthcare costs in the long run. By preventing or managing chronic diseases associated with obesity, you can avoid expensive medical treatments and interventions.

Chapter 1: The Benefits of Weight Loss

Increased Energy Levels

Carrying excess weight can leave you feeling sluggish and fatigued. The strain on your body makes it harder to move and engage in physical activities, leading to a sedentary lifestyle and a lack of energy. However, losing weight can bring about a significant increase in energy levels.

When you shed those extra pounds, your body becomes more efficient at using energy, and your metabolism improves. This means you'll have more energy to carry out daily tasks and participate in physical activities. With increased energy levels, you'll find it easier to engage in exercise and enjoy a more active lifestyle.

Whether it's going for a run, playing sports, or simply taking a walk, you'll have the energy and stamina to participate in activities that bring you joy and improve your overall fitness. Additionally, having higher energy levels can positively impact your productivity and focus throughout the day, leading to increased success in both personal and professional endeavors.

Enhanced Mood and Mental Well-being

Weight loss has a significant impact on mood and mental well-being. Achieving a healthy weight can boost your self-confidence and improve your body image, leading to a positive effect on your overall mood and self-esteem.

Losing weight can also reduce symptoms of depression and anxiety. Exercise releases endorphins, known as "feel-good" hormones that elevate your mood and reduce feelings of stress and anxiety. By engaging in regular physical activity as part of your weight loss journey, you can experience these mood-boosting benefits.

Furthermore, achieving a healthy weight can lead to improved mental clarity and cognitive function. Proper nutrition and regular exercise support brain health, helping you think more clearly and improve your focus and memory.

Overall, losing weight can have a transformative effect on your mental well-being. It can increase your self-confidence, reduce symptoms of depression and anxiety, and improve your overall mood and mental clarity.

Remember that weight loss is a journey, and it's important to approach it with patience and a focus on overall well-being. By adopting healthy habits and making sustainable lifestyle changes, you can experience the numerous benefits that come with achieving a healthy weight.

Setting Realistic Weight Loss Goals

Setting realistic weight loss goals is an essential step in your weight loss journey. It's important to have a clear understanding of what is achievable and safe for your body. When setting your weight loss objectives, keep the following important factors in mind:

1. Assess Your Current Health Status: Before setting weight loss goals, it's

crucial to assess your current health status. This includes factors such as your body mass index (BMI), blood pressure, cholesterol levels, and any underlying health conditions you may have. Understanding your starting point can help you set realistic goals that are appropriate for your individual circumstances.

2. Consider Your Lifestyle: Take into account your lifestyle and daily commitments when setting weight loss goals. Consider factors such as your work schedule, family responsibilities, and social activities. It's important to set goals that are realistic and sustainable within the context of your lifestyle.

3. Gradual and Sustainable Approach: Aim for gradual and sustainable weight loss rather than quick fixes or

drastic measures. Most people agree that losing 1-2 pounds each week is a good and doable goal. Muscle loss, vitamin shortages, and rebound weight gain are frequently consequences of rapid weight reduction.

4. Focus on Health, Not Just Numbers: Instead of solely focusing on the number on the scale, shift your focus to improving your overall health. Set goals that include other markers of progress such as increased energy levels, improved sleep quality, reduced waist circumference, or improved fitness levels.

5. Break it Down into Smaller Goals: Break your overall weight loss goal into smaller, more manageable milestones. You may use this to monitor your progress and maintain motivation. Celebrating these smaller

victories can boost your confidence and keep you motivated to continue working towards your ultimate goal.

6. Be Realistic and Flexible: Set goals that are realistic for you and take into account any potential challenges or setbacks that may arise. Weight loss is not always a linear process, and it's important to be flexible and adapt your goals as needed. Remember that progress is not always measured by the number on the scale but by the positive changes you make in your lifestyle and habits.

7. Seek Support: Consider seeking support from a healthcare professional, registered dietitian, or weight loss support group. They can provide guidance, accountability, and motivation throughout your weight loss journey.

Chapter 2: Nutrition and weight loss

When it comes to weight loss, diet plays a crucial role in achieving and maintaining a healthy body weight. we will now delve into the significance of a well-balanced diet in weight loss, highlighting its impact on calorie intake, nutrient quality, and overall success in achieving weight loss goals.

1. Calorie Intake and Energy Balance:

Weight loss is primarily determined by the balance between calorie intake and energy expenditure. It is imperative to consume fewer calories than the body expels in order to lose weight.. A well-designed diet can help create a calorie deficit by providing adequate nutrition while reducing excessive calorie intake. By focusing on portion control and making healthier food choices, individuals can effectively manage their calorie intake and promote weight loss.

2. Nutrient Quality and Satiety:

A healthy diet for weight loss should not only focus on calorie reduction but also prioritize nutrient quality. Consuming nutrient-dense foods, such as fruits, vegetables, lean proteins, whole grains, and healthy fats, provides essential vitamins, minerals, and fiber while promoting satiety. These foods help individuals feel full for longer periods, reducing the likelihood of overeating and aiding in weight loss efforts.

3. Balancing Macronutrients:

The distribution of macronutrients (carbohydrates, proteins, and fats) in a diet can significantly impact weight loss. A balanced diet should include an appropriate ratio of these macronutrients to support overall health and weight management. For example, a diet rich in lean proteins can help preserve muscle mass, which is crucial for maintaining a healthy metabolism during weight loss. Additionally, incorporating healthy fats and complex carbohydrates can provide sustained energy and promote dietary adherence.

4. Building Healthy Eating Habits:

Successful weight loss involves adopting healthy eating habits that can be sustained in the long term. Crash diets or extreme restrictions are often unsustainable and can lead to weight regain. Instead, focusing on portion control, mindful eating, and incorporating a variety of nutritious foods can help individuals develop a healthy relationship with food and make lasting lifestyle changes.

5. Seeking Professional Guidance:

While making dietary changes for weight loss, it is advisable to seek guidance from healthcare professionals or registered dietitians. These experts can provide personalized recommendations based on individual needs, goals, and any underlying health conditions. They can also help individuals navigate through conflicting information and develop a sustainable and effective weight loss plan.

Foods to include in your weight loss diet

Fruits and Vegetables

Your best friends when it comes to weight loss, are fruits and vegetables. They are low in calories, high in fiber, and packed with essential vitamins, minerals, and antioxidants. Including a variety of fruits and vegetables in your diet can help you feel full, satisfied, and nourished. Here are some fruits and vegetables that you should include in your weight loss diet:

1. Berries:
Berries like strawberries, blueberries, raspberries, and blackberries are not only delicious but also low in calories and high in antioxidants. They are rich in fiber, which aids in digestion

and helps control hunger. Add them to your breakfast cereal, yogurt, or enjoy them as a snack.

2. Leafy Greens:
Leafy greens such as spinach, kale, Swiss chard, and arugula are excellent choices for weight loss. They contain lots of vitamins and minerals, have few calories, and are high in fiber. Incorporate them into salads, stir-fries, or smoothies for a nutritious boost.

3. Cruciferous Vegetables:
Cruciferous vegetables like broccoli, cauliflower, Brussels sprouts, and cabbage are not only nutritious but also low in calories. They are rich in fiber and contain compounds that may help support weight loss. Steam, roast, or stir-fry them to enjoy their benefits.

4. Citrus Fruits:
Citrus fruits like oranges, grapefruits, lemons, and limes are refreshing and packed with vitamin C. They are low in calories and high in fiber, making them a great addition to your weight loss diet. Enjoy them as a snack, in salads, or squeeze them into water for a refreshing drink.

5. Apples:
Apples are high in fiber and water content, making them a filling and satisfying fruit for weight loss. They also contain antioxidants and are a great source of natural sweetness. Enjoy them as a snack, slice them into salads, or add them to your oatmeal.

6. Carrots:
Carrots are fibrous, calorie-efficient, and crisp. They are also packed with beta-carotene, which is converted into vitamin A in the body.

Incorporate carrots into your salads, stir-fries, or enjoy them as a snack with hummus or a healthy dip.

7. Bell Peppers:
Bell peppers come in various colors and are packed with vitamins A and C. They are low in calories and high in fiber, making them a great addition to your weight loss diet. Include them in stir-fries, salads, or stuff them with lean protein for a nutritious meal.

Remember to aim for a variety of fruits and vegetables to benefit from their different nutrients. Experiment with different cooking methods and recipes to keep your meals exciting and enjoyable.

Whole Grains and Legumes

Whole grains and legumes are excellent additions to a weight loss diet. They are rich in fiber, protein, and essential nutrients, making them filling and satisfying. Including these foods can help control hunger, stabilize blood sugar levels, and promote healthy digestion. Here are some whole grains and legumes that you should include in your weight loss diet:

1. Brown Rice:
Brown rice is a whole grain that is high in fiber and provides sustained energy. Since it keeps the nutrient-rich bran and germ layers, it is a healthier option to white rice.. Use brown rice as a base for stir-fries, salads, or as a side dish to accompany lean protein.

2. Quinoa:
Quinoa is a versatile grain that is packed with protein, fiber, and essential amino acids. It is gluten-free and has a nutty flavor. Use quinoa as a substitute for rice or pasta, or add it to salads for a nutritious boost.

3. Oats:
Oats are a great source of soluble fiber, which helps you feel full and satisfied. They are also rich in antioxidants and can help lower cholesterol levels. Enjoy a bowl of oatmeal for breakfast or use oats in baking healthy treats like granola bars or cookies.

4. Whole Wheat Bread:
To improve your intake of fiber, use whole wheat bread instead of refined white bread. Whole wheat bread is made from whole grains, which provide more nutrients and fiber. Use

it to make sandwiches or toast, and choose options with minimal added sugars or preservatives.

5. Lentils:
Lentils are legumes that are high in protein, fiber, and complex carbohydrates. They come in various colors, such as green, brown, and red, and can be used in soups, stews, salads, or as a side dish. Lentils are a great vegetarian source of protein and can help you feel full for longer.

6. Chickpeas:
Chickpeas, also known as garbanzo beans, are versatile legumes that are rich in fiber, protein, and essential minerals. They may be roasted for a crispy snack, added to salads, or used to create hummus. Chickpeas are a great plant-based protein source and can be incorporated into various dishes.

7. Black Beans:
Black beans are another legume that is high in fiber and protein. They are also a good source of iron, antioxidants, and folate. Use black beans in recipes such as soups, stews, tacos, or salads for a nutritious and satisfying meal.

Remember to cook whole grains and legumes properly to enhance their digestibility and nutrient availability. Soak legumes before cooking to reduce cooking time and improve their texture. By including these whole grains and legumes in your weight loss diet, you'll not only nourish your body but also support your weight loss goals.

Including lean protein sources in your weight loss diet is essential for building and maintaining muscle mass, promoting satiety, and supporting overall health. Lean proteins are low in fat and calories, making them an ideal choice for weight loss. Here are some lean protein sources that you should include in your diet:

1. Chicken Breast:
Chicken breast is a lean protein option that is low in fat and high in protein. It is versatile and can be grilled, baked, or sautéed. Remove the skin to reduce the fat content further and enjoy it as part of a salad, stir-fry, or as the main protein in a meal.

2. Turkey:

Turkey is another lean protein source that is low in fat and rich in protein. It can be used as a substitute for chicken in various recipes. Ground turkey can be used to make burgers, meatballs, or added to chili for a satisfying meal.

3. Fish:

Fish, such as salmon, tuna, trout, and cod, are excellent sources of lean protein and omega-3 fatty acids. Omega-3 fatty acids have been shown to support weight loss and reduce inflammation. Grill, bake, or steam fish for a healthy and delicious meal.

4. Tofu:

Low in calories and high in protein, tofu is a plant-based source of protein. It is a versatile ingredient that can be used in stir-fries, salads, or as a substitute for meat in various dishes. Tofu absorbs flavors well, making it a great addition to your weight loss diet.

5. Tempeh:
Tempeh is another plant-based protein source that is made from fermented soybeans.It has a lot of minerals, fiber, and protein. Use tempeh in stir-fries, sandwiches, or marinate and grill it for a tasty and nutritious meal.

6. Lentils and Chickpeas:
Lentils and chickpeas are not only excellent sources of fiber and complex carbohydrates but also provide a good amount of protein. They are versatile and can be used in soups, stews, salads, or as a side dish. Incorporating lentils and chickpeas into your diet can add variety and nutritional value.

7. Greek Yogurt:

Greek yogurt is a creamy and tangy protein source that is low in fat and high in calcium. It can be enjoyed as a snack, added to smoothies, or used as a substitute for sour cream or mayonnaise in recipes. Choose plain, unsweetened Greek yogurt to avoid added sugars.

Healthy fats and oils

When it comes to weight loss, it's important to include healthy fats and oils in your diet. Not all fats, despite popular belief, are unhealthy for you. In fact, incorporating the right types of fats into your meals can actually support your weight loss efforts. Here are some examples of healthy fats and oils to include in your weight loss diet:

1. Avocado: Avocados are a great source of monounsaturated fats, which have been shown to promote satiety and help control appetite. They are also packed with fiber, vitamins, and minerals, making them a nutritious addition to any meal.

2. Olive oil: Olive oil is rich in monounsaturated fats and contains antioxidants that have been linked to various health benefits, including weight loss. It can be used as a dressing for salads or as a cooking oil for sautéing vegetables.

3. Nuts and seeds: Nuts and seeds: Excellent sources of good fats include almonds, walnuts, chia seeds, and flaxseeds. They also provide a good amount of protein and fiber, which can help keep you feeling full and satisfied.

4. Coconut oil: Coconut oil contains medium-chain triglycerides (MCTs), which are easily digested and can be used as a quick source of energy. It has been shown to speed up metabolism and encourage fat burning.

5. Fatty fish: Fish like salmon, mackerel, and sardines are high in omega-3 fatty acids, which have been associated with numerous health benefits, including weight loss. Omega-3s can help reduce inflammation, improve insulin sensitivity, and support a healthy metabolism.

6. Seeds: Seeds such as pumpkin seeds, sunflower seeds, and sesame seeds are rich in healthy fats and provide a good amount of fiber and protein. They can be sprinkled on

salads, yogurt, or added to smoothies for an extra nutritional boost.

Low calorie snacks and desserts

When it comes to weight loss, finding low-calorie snacks and desserts can be a game-changer. These options allow you to satisfy your cravings without derailing your progress. Here are some ideas for low-calorie snacks and desserts to include in your weight loss diet:

1. Greek yogurt with berries: Greek yogurt is high in protein and low in calories, making it an excellent choice for a satisfying snack. Top it with a handful of fresh berries for added flavor and antioxidants.

2. Veggie sticks with hummus: Cut up some carrots, cucumbers, and bell peppers and pair them with a serving of hummus. This combination provides a

good amount of fiber and nutrients while keeping the calorie count low.

3. Air-popped popcorn: Popcorn is a great low-calorie snack option as long as it's not drenched in butter or excessive amounts of salt. Opt for air-popped popcorn and season it with herbs or spices for a flavorful treat.

4. Frozen grapes: Freeze a bunch of grapes for a refreshing and sweet snack. They offer a satisfying crunch and can help curb your sweet tooth without adding many calories.

5. Chia seed pudding: Mix chia seeds with unsweetened almond milk or coconut milk and let it sit overnight. The chia seeds will absorb the liquid and create a pudding-like texture that is rich in fiber and omega-3 fatty acids.

6. Dark chocolate: Choose dark chocolate with a high cocoa content (70% or more) for a guilt-free dessert option. It contains antioxidants and can satisfy your chocolate cravings without the excess sugar and calories found in milk chocolate.

7. Apple slices with nut butter: Slice up an apple and pair it with a tablespoon of your favorite nut butter, such as almond or peanut butter. This combination offers a balance of fiber, healthy fats, and protein.

8. Rice cake with avocado: Spread mashed avocado on a rice cake for a crunchy and satisfying snack. Avocado provides healthy fats, while the rice cake keeps the calorie count low.

Foods to limit or avoid for weight loss

High-fat dairy products:

High-fat dairy products like whole milk, cheese, and butter should be limited or avoided when trying to lose weight. These products are high in saturated fats and calories, which can contribute to weight gain and other health issues. Instead, opt for lower-fat alternatives like skim milk, reduced-fat cheese, or Greek yogurt.

Saturated fats are known to raise cholesterol levels and increase the risk of heart disease. By choosing lower-fat dairy options, you can reduce your intake of saturated fats and promote a healthier heart.

Additionally, high-fat dairy products tend to be calorie-dense, meaning they contain a significant amount of calories in a small serving size. This can make it easy to consume excess calories without feeling satisfied. By choosing lower-fat options, you can enjoy dairy products while keeping your calorie intake in check.

Highly processed and refined grains:

Foods made with refined grains like white bread, white rice, and pasta should be limited or avoided for weight loss. These foods have been stripped of their fiber and nutrients during processing, leaving behind empty calories that can spike blood sugar levels and lead to weight gain.

Refined grains also tend to be low in fiber, which is important for promoting feelings of fullness and reducing hunger. Without adequate fiber, you may find yourself feeling hungry soon after consuming refined grain products, leading to overeating and potential weight gain.

Instead of refined grains, choose whole grain options like whole wheat bread, brown rice, quinoa, or whole grain pasta. Whole grains retain their fiber and nutrients, providing a more filling and nutritious choice. They also have a lower glycemic index, meaning they have a slower impact on blood sugar levels and can help keep you satisfied for longer periods.

Sugary desserts:

Sugary desserts like cakes, cookies, ice cream, and pastries should be limited or avoided when trying to lose weight. These treats are often high in added sugars and unhealthy fats, making them calorie-dense and lacking in nutritional value.

Consuming excessive amounts of added sugars can lead to weight gain and increase the risk of chronic diseases like obesity, type 2 diabetes, and heart disease. By reducing your intake of sugary desserts, you can lower your overall sugar consumption and support weight loss efforts.

Instead of completely depriving yourself of desserts, try healthier alternatives like fruit salads, yogurt with berries, or homemade treats using natural sweeteners like dates or honey. These options provide natural sweetness and additional nutrients, making them a more nutritious choice for satisfying your sweet tooth while still supporting your weight loss goals.

Chapter 3: Exercise and physical activity for weight loss

Exercise and physical activity play a crucial role in weight loss and overall health. Incorporating regular exercise into your routine can help you burn calories, build muscle, improve cardiovascular health, and boost metabolism. Here are some key points to consider when it comes to exercise and physical activity for weight loss:

The Importance of Exercise in Weight Loss:

Exercise is very important for any weight loss journey. It helps create an energy deficit, which is necessary for losing weight. When you engage in physical activity, your body burns calories, and when you burn more calories than you consume, you create a calorie deficit, leading to weight loss.

Exercise also helps increase muscle mass. As you engage in strength training exercises, your muscles adapt and become stronger. This increase in muscle mass not only helps you burn more calories during exercise but also increases your resting metabolic rate. Muscle burns more calories at rest than fat, so having more muscle can boost your metabolism and aid in weight loss.

Regular exercise also has numerous benefits for cardiovascular health. Cardiovascular exercises, such as running, cycling, swimming, or brisk walking, help improve heart health by strengthening the heart muscle and improving blood flow. These exercises increase heart rate and help burn calories, contributing to weight loss.

Exercise is crucial for mental health as well as physical health. Physical activity releases endorphins, which are known as "feel-good" hormones. These endorphins can improve mood, reduce stress and anxiety, and enhance overall mental well-being. This can be especially beneficial during a weight loss journey, as it can help combat any negative emotions or stress associated with the process.

Incorporating exercise into your weight loss plan also helps with weight maintenance. Regular physical activity can help prevent weight regain by increasing muscle mass and maintaining a higher metabolic rate. It also helps improve body composition by reducing fat mass and preserving lean muscle mass.

Overall, exercise is a vital component of weight loss. It helps create a calorie deficit, increases muscle mass and metabolism, improves cardiovascular health, enhances mental well-being, and aids in weight maintenance. By incorporating regular exercise into your routine, you can optimize your weight loss efforts and improve your overall health.

Types of Exercises for Weight Loss:

Cardiovascular Exercises:

Cardiovascular exercises, also known as aerobic exercises, are an excellent choice for weight loss. These exercises elevate your heart rate and increase calorie burn, helping you create a calorie deficit. Some popular cardiovascular exercises include:

- Running or Jogging: Running or jogging is a high-intensity exercise that can help burn a significant number of calories. It can be done outdoors or on a treadmill, making it accessible to almost everyone.

- Cycling: Cycling can be done outdoors or on a stationary bike as it is a low-impact exercise. It not only burns calories but also strengthens the lower body muscles.

- Swimming: Swimming is a full-body exercise that works a variety of muscle groups. It is a low-impact exercise that is gentle on the joints, making it suitable for individuals with joint issues.

- Brisk Walking: Brisk walking is a simple yet effective exercise for weight loss. It can be easily incorporated into your daily routine and can be done anywhere, making it accessible to all fitness levels.

- Dancing: A pleasant and entertaining approach to burn calories is through dancing. Whether it's Zumba, hip-hop, or salsa, dancing can help you shed pounds while having a great time.

Strength Training Exercises:

Strength training exercises are crucial for weight loss as they help build lean muscle mass. More muscle means a higher resting metabolic rate, which leads to increased calorie burn even at rest. below are some examples of strength training exercises:

- Weightlifting: Weightlifting involves using free weights or weight machines to target specific muscle groups. Strength, muscular mass, and general body composition are all improved.

- Bodyweight Exercises: Bodyweight exercises, such as push-ups, squats, lunges, and planks, use your body weight as resistance. These exercises can be done anywhere without any equipment and are effective in building muscle and burning calories.

- Resistance Band Workouts: Resistance bands are portable and versatile tools that can be used for strength training exercises. They provide resistance throughout the movement, helping to build muscle and increase calorie burn.

High-Intensity Interval Training (HIIT):

High-Intensity Interval Training (HIIT) is a form of exercise that alternates between short bursts of intense activity and periods of rest or low-intensity activity. HIIT exercises are renowned for being effective in burning fat and calories. Some examples of HIIT exercises include:

- Burpees: Burpees are a full-body workout that consists of a squat, push-up, and jump. They are highly effective in raising your heart rate and burning calories.

- Jumping Jacks: Jumping jacks are a simple yet effective exercise that gets your heart rate up. They work a variety of muscle areas and can be done anywhere.

- Mountain Climbers: Mountain climbers target the core, arms, and legs. They involve bringing your knees towards your chest while in a plank position, simulating climbing a mountain.

- High-Knee Running: Running while raising your knees as high as you can is known as high-knee running. It is an intense exercise that engages the core, glutes, and leg muscles.

Incorporating a combination of cardiovascular exercises, strength training exercises, and HIIT workouts into your routine can help maximize weight loss and improve overall fitness levels. It is important to consult with a healthcare professional or certified trainer before starting any new exercise program to ensure it is suitable for your individual needs and abilities.

Creating a Personalized Exercise Plan:

Creating a personalized exercise plan is essential for achieving weight loss goals effectively and safely. Here are some steps to help you create a plan that suits your individual needs:

1. Set Specific Goals: Determine your weight loss goals and establish a timeline for achieving them. Make sure your goals are realistic and achievable.

2. Assess Your Current Fitness Level: Evaluate your current fitness level to determine your starting point. Consider factors such as cardiovascular endurance, strength, flexibility, and overall health.

3. Choose the Right Exercises: Based on your goals and fitness level, select a combination of cardiovascular exercises, strength training exercises, and HIIT workouts that you enjoy and are suitable for your abilities. Consider incorporating a variety of exercises to keep your workouts interesting and challenging.

4. Determine Frequency and Duration: Decide how often you will exercise and for how long. Aim for at least 150 minutes of moderate-intensity cardio exercise per week, along with two or more days of strength training exercises. As your fitness level advances, gradually increase the length and intensity of your workouts.

5. Create a Schedule: Plan your exercise sessions in advance and schedule them into your weekly

routine. Consider them to be appointments you must keep with yourself.

6. Warm-Up and Cool-Down: Prioritize warm-up exercises to prepare your body for the workout and cool-down exercises to gradually bring your heart rate down and prevent muscle soreness.

7. Monitor Progress: Keep track of your workouts, noting the exercises performed, duration, intensity, and any improvements or challenges you encounter. Regularly assess your progress to stay motivated and make necessary adjustments to your plan.

8. Listen to Your Body: Pay attention to how your body feels during and after exercise. If you encounter discomfort or pain, change your workout or stop altogether. It's

important to prioritize safety and avoid pushing yourself beyond your limits.

9. Stay Consistent: Consistency is key to achieving weight loss goals. Stick to your exercise plan even on days when you may not feel motivated. Keep in mind that every workout counts towards your success.

10. Seek Professional Guidance: If you're unsure about designing an exercise plan or need assistance, consider consulting with a healthcare professional or certified trainer. They can provide personalized guidance, tailor exercises to your specific needs, and ensure you're on the right track.

Chapter 4: Behavior and Lifestyle Changes for Weight Loss Success

Mindful Eating and Portion Control:

Being totally present and attentive when you eat is a key component of the mindful eating technique. By practicing mindful eating, you can develop a healthier relationship with food and improve portion control. Here are some strategies to incorporate mindful eating and portion control into your weight loss journey:

1. Eat slowly: Take your time to chew each bite thoroughly and savor the flavors of your food. Eating slowly allows your brain to register feelings of fullness, preventing overeating.

2. Use smaller plates and bowls: Opt for smaller plates and bowls to visually trick your brain into perceiving larger portions. You may feel fuller after eating less as a result of this.

3. Pay attention to hunger and fullness cues: Before eating, assess your level of hunger on a scale from 1 to 10. Aim to start eating when you are moderately hungry (around a 3 or 4) and stop when you feel comfortably full (around a 6 or 7). Listen to your body's signals and avoid mindless eating.

4. Practice portion control: Learn to estimate appropriate portion sizes for different food groups. Use visual cues, such as comparing serving sizes to everyday objects (e.g., a deck of cards for meat) or using measuring cups

and spoons until you become more familiar with appropriate portions.

5. Take breaks during meals: Pause halfway through your meal to assess your level of hunger and fullness. This allows you to gauge if you need more food or if you're satisfied and can stop eating.

6. Avoid emotional eating: Be mindful of the emotional cues that might cause binge eating. Instead of turning to food for comfort, find alternative ways to cope with emotions, such as journaling, going for a walk, or talking to a supportive friend.

7. Practice gratitude: Before starting your meal, take a moment to appreciate the food in front of you. Acknowledge the effort that went into preparing it and the nourishment it provides for your body.

8. Engage your senses: Notice the colors, smells, textures, and flavors of your food. Engaging your senses can enhance your eating experience and increase satisfaction with smaller portions.

9. Stay hydrated: Drink water throughout your meal to help you feel fuller and prevent overeating. Sip water between bites to slow down your eating pace.

10. Reflect on your eating experience: After each meal, take a moment to reflect on how you feel physically and emotionally. Assess whether you ate mindfully and if there are any adjustments you can make for future meals.

Meal Planning and Preparation Tips:

Meal planning and preparation can be instrumental in achieving weight loss success. You may choose healthier options, manage portion sizes, and prevent impulsive eating by planning and preparing your meals in advance. Here are some tips for effective meal planning and preparation:

1. Set aside time for meal planning: Dedicate a specific time each week to plan your meals. This can be done on a Sunday or any other convenient day. Consider your schedule, dietary preferences, and nutritional needs when selecting recipes.

2. Create a balanced meal plan: Aim to include a variety of nutrient-dense foods in your meal plan, such as lean

proteins, whole grains, fruits, vegetables, and healthy fats. Ensure that your meals are well-balanced and provide all the necessary nutrients.

3. Make a shopping list: Once you have planned your meals, create a shopping list based on the ingredients you will need. Stick to your list while grocery shopping to avoid purchasing unhealthy or unnecessary items.

4. Prepare meals in advance: Take advantage of your free time to prepare meals in advance. Cook larger batches of food and portion them out into individual containers for easy grab-and-go options throughout the week. This can help you avoid relying on unhealthy takeout or fast food when you're busy or tired.

5. Use time-saving kitchen tools: Invest in kitchen tools that can help streamline your meal preparation process. For example, a slow cooker or Instant Pot can be used to cook large quantities of food with minimal effort.

6. Pack healthy snacks: Prepare healthy snacks in advance and portion them into snack-sized bags or containers. This way, you'll have nutritious options readily available when hunger strikes between meals.

7. Have a backup plan: Life can be unpredictable, so it's important to have a backup plan for those days when you don't have time to cook or forgot to bring your prepared meals. Keep some healthy frozen meals, canned soups, or pre-cut vegetables on hand as convenient alternatives.

8. Stay organized: Keep your pantry, refrigerator, and freezer well-organized to easily locate ingredients and prevent food waste. To make sure you eat the prepared meals before they go bad, label and date them.

9. Get creative with leftovers: Don't throw away any leftovers. Repurpose them into new meals or use them as components for salads or wraps. By doing this, you may save time and money while still getting to eat scrumptious meals.

10. Be flexible: Remember that meal planning is not set in stone. Be open to adjusting your plan based on your changing needs or preferences. Allow room for spontaneity and enjoy dining out or trying new recipes occasionally.

Strategies for Overcoming Emotional Eating:

Emotional eating refers to the tendency to eat in response to emotions rather than physical hunger. It can often lead to overeating and hinder weight loss progress. Here are some methods for avoiding emotional eating:

1. Identify triggers: Pay attention to the emotions, situations, or events that trigger your emotional eating episodes. You may be able to anticipate and get ready for certain triggers with the use of this knowledge.

2. Find alternative coping mechanisms: Instead of turning to food for comfort, find alternative ways to cope with emotions. Engage in activities that bring you joy, such

as reading, listening to music, practicing mindfulness or deep breathing exercises, taking a bath, or engaging in a hobby.

3. Practice mindful eating: As mentioned earlier, practice mindful eating by paying attention to your eating habits and being fully present during meals. You may use this to distinguish between actual hunger and emotional desires.

4. Keep a food journal: Maintain a food journal to track your eating patterns and identify any emotional triggers or patterns. You should record your food intake, eating times, and feelings both before and after meals. This can help you identify patterns and make connections between your emotions and eating behaviors.

5. Seek support: Reach out to a trusted friend, family member, or therapist who can provide emotional support and guidance. Talking about your emotions and struggles with someone who understands can be helpful in overcoming emotional eating.

6. Practice stress management techniques: Find healthy ways to manage stress, as stress often triggers emotional eating. Engage in activities such as exercise, yoga, meditation, or deep breathing exercises to help reduce stress levels.

7. Create a supportive environment: Surround yourself with a supportive environment that promotes healthy eating habits. Remove tempting or triggering foods from your home and stock it with nutritious options instead.

8. Practice self-compassion: Be kind to yourself and avoid self-judgment when you experience emotional eating episodes. Understand that it is a common struggle and focus on learning from the experience rather than dwelling on it.

9. Develop healthy coping strategies: Experiment with different coping strategies to find what works best for you. Be patient with yourself since it could take some time to find healthier alternatives to eating to cope with emotions.

10. Seek professional help if needed: If emotional eating is significantly impacting your well-being or ability to manage your weight, consider seeking professional help from a registered dietitian, therapist, or counselor who specializes in

emotional eating or disordered eating behaviors.

Managing Stress and Sleep for Weight Loss:

Weight loss attempts can be significantly impacted by stress and sleep deprivation. Both can disrupt hormone levels, increase cravings for unhealthy foods, and hinder the body's ability to burn fat efficiently. Here are some strategies for managing stress and improving sleep to support weight loss:

1. Prioritize self-care: Make taking care of yourself a top priority each day. Engage in activities that help you relax and unwind, such as taking a bath, reading a book, practicing yoga or meditation, or spending time in nature.

2. Exercise regularly: Regular physical activity can help reduce stress levels and improve sleep quality. Aim for at least 150 minutes per week of strength training and moderate-intensity aerobic activity.

3. Practice stress management techniques: Find stress management techniques that work for you, such as deep breathing exercises, mindfulness meditation, progressive muscle relaxation, or engaging in a hobby you enjoy. Experiment with different techniques to find what helps you relax and reduce stress.

4. Get enough sleep: Attempt to get 7-9 hours of good sleep each night. Create a relaxing bedtime routine, ensure your sleep environment is comfortable and free from

distractions, and establish a consistent sleep schedule.

5. Limit caffeine and alcohol intake: Both caffeine and alcohol can disrupt sleep patterns and increase stress levels. Limit your intake of these substances, especially in the evening, to promote better sleep and reduce stress.

6. Establish boundaries: Learn to say no to excessive commitments or obligations that may contribute to stress. Set boundaries to protect your time and prioritize activities that are important for your well-being.

7. Seek social support: Surround yourself with a supportive network of friends and family who can provide emotional support during times of stress. Share your concerns and seek their guidance when needed.

8. Practice relaxation techniques: Incorporate relaxation techniques into your daily routine to help manage stress levels. Deep breathing techniques, gradual muscular relaxation, guided visualization, and relaxing music are some examples of this.

9. Consider therapy or counseling: If stress is significantly impacting your life and weight loss efforts, consider seeking professional help from a therapist or counselor who specializes in stress management techniques.

10. Take breaks and practice self-reflection: Regularly take breaks throughout the day to recharge and reflect on your stress levels. Use this time to engage in activities that bring you joy or to assess any potential

sources of stress that can be addressed.

Chapter 5: tracking progress and staying motivated

Tracking Progress:

One way to stay motivated on your weight loss journey is by tracking your progress. This can help you see the positive changes you're making and keep you motivated to continue. below are ways to track your progress:

- Keep a food journal: Write down everything you eat and drink throughout the day. This might assist you in being more conscious of your eating patterns and selecting healthier options. You can also track your calorie intake and macronutrient breakdown if that's something you're interested in.

- Use a fitness tracker: Invest in a fitness tracker or use a smartphone app to track your daily activity levels. This can include steps taken, calories burned, and even sleep patterns. Seeing your progress in terms of increased activity can be motivating and encourage you to keep moving.

- Take measurements: Along with weighing yourself, take measurements of your body, such as waist circumference, hip circumference, and thigh circumference. This can help you see changes in your body shape even if the scale doesn't budge. Remember that muscle weighs more than fat, so you may be losing inches even if the number on the scale doesn't change much.

- Take progress photos: Take photos of yourself at the start of your weight loss journey and then periodically throughout. Seeing the physical changes in your body can be incredibly motivating and remind you of how far you've come.

Setting Goals:

Setting realistic and achievable goals is essential for staying motivated on your weight loss journey. below are tips for setting goals:

- Make them specific: Instead of setting a vague goal like "lose weight," make it more specific, such as "lose 10 pounds in 2 months" or "fit into my favorite pair of jeans comfortably."

- Make them measurable: Set goals that can be measured, such as tracking your progress through pounds lost, inches lost, or body fat percentage. Having a measurable goal allows you to track your progress and see how far you've come.

- Make them realistic: Set goals that are realistic and attainable. Losing 1-2 pounds per week is considered a healthy and achievable rate of weight loss. Setting unattainable objectives might sap your drive by causing you to feel frustrated and disappointed.

- Break them down: Break your larger weight loss goal into smaller, more manageable goals. For example, if your overall goal is to lose 50 pounds, set smaller goals of losing 5 pounds at a time. Achieving these smaller goals along the way can help keep you motivated.

Celebrate Milestones:

Celebrating milestones along your weight loss journey can provide a sense of accomplishment and keep you motivated to continue. Here are some ways to celebrate your achievements:

- Treat yourself: When you reach a milestone, treat yourself to something non-food related that you enjoy. This could be buying a new workout outfit, getting a massage, or taking a day off work to relax and recharge.

- Share your success: Inform your loved ones who are helping you on your weight loss journey about your accomplishments. They can provide encouragement and celebrate your success with you.

- Reward yourself with a healthy indulgence: Instead of reaching for unhealthy treats to celebrate, reward yourself with a healthy indulgence. This could be trying a new healthy recipe, going for a hike in nature, or taking a fitness class you've been wanting to try.

- Reflect on your progress: Take some time to reflect on how far you've come and the positive changes you've made. Write down a list of all the accomplishments you've achieved so far and remind yourself of them when you need an extra boost of motivation.

Stay Accountable:

Staying accountable to your weight loss goals can help you stay motivated and on track. To maintain accountability, try the following:

- Find a weight loss buddy: Join forces with a relative or acquaintance who shares your objectives. Check in with each other regularly to share progress, provide support, and hold each other accountable.

- Join a weight loss support group: Consider joining a weight loss support group or online community where you can connect with others who are on a similar journey. Share your successes, challenges, and tips with each other to stay motivated.

- Hire a personal trainer or nutritionist: If you need extra support and accountability, consider hiring a professional to help guide you on your weight loss journey. They can provide personalized advice, create a tailored workout plan, and help you stay motivated.

- Use technology: There are many apps and websites available that can help you track your progress, set goals, and provide motivation. Utilize these tools to stay accountable and keep track of your progress.

Chapter 6: sustainable weight loss and maintenance

Creating Healthy Habits:

One of the keys to sustainable weight loss and maintenance is creating healthy habits. below are tips for developing healthy habits:

- Make small, gradual changes: Instead of trying to overhaul your entire lifestyle overnight, start by making small, manageable changes. For example, swap out sugary drinks for water, incorporate more fruits and vegetables into your meals, or take the stairs instead of the elevator.

- Focus on balance: Aim for a varied, nutrient-dense diet that is well-balanced. Your meals should contain lean proteins, whole grains, fruits, veggies, and healthy fats. Avoid labeling foods as "good" or "bad" and instead focus on moderation and portion control.

- Prioritize physical activity: Find activities that you enjoy and make them a regular part of your routine. Aim for at least 150 minutes of moderate-intensity aerobic activity or 75 minutes of vigorous-intensity activity each week, along with strength training exercises at least twice a week.

- Practice mindful eating: Pay heed to your body's signs for hunger and fullness. Eat slowly and savor each bite, focusing on the taste, texture, and enjoyment of the food. Keep your attention off of other things when eating, such as watching TV or going through your phone.

- Get enough sleep: Your hormones might be upset by sleep deprivation, which increases your desire for unhealthy meals. Aim for 7-9 hours of quality sleep each night to support your weight loss and overall health.

Building a Support System:

Having a strong support system can greatly contribute to sustainable weight loss and maintenance. Here are some ways to build a support system:

- Enlist the help of friends and family: Share your goals with your loved ones and ask for their support. They can provide encouragement, accountability, and join you in making healthier choices.

- Join a weight loss program or support group: Consider joining a weight loss program or support group where you can connect with others who are on a similar journey. These groups often provide valuable resources, tips, and motivation.

- Seek professional help: If you're struggling to reach your weight loss goals or maintain your progress, consider seeking the help of a registered dietitian, therapist, or weight loss coach. They can provide personalized guidance and support.

- Find online communities: There are many online communities and forums dedicated to weight loss and healthy living. Joining these communities can provide a sense of belonging, support, and motivation.

Managing Stress and Emotional Eating:

Weight loss efforts can frequently be sabotaged by stress and emotional eating. below are a few techniques for preventing stress and emotional eating:

- Identify triggers: Pay attention to what makes you anxious or causes you to overeat. It could be certain situations, emotions, or even specific foods. Once you identify your triggers, you can develop strategies to cope with them in healthier ways.

- Find alternative coping mechanisms: Instead of turning to food when stressed or emotional, find alternative coping mechanisms that help you relax and unwind. This could include practicing deep breathing exercises, going for a walk, listening to music, or journaling.

- Practice self-care: Prioritize self-care activities that help reduce stress and promote emotional well-being. This could include taking a bath, practicing yoga or meditation, getting a massage, or engaging in hobbies you enjoy.

- Seek support: Reach out to friends, family, or a therapist for support when you're feeling stressed or overwhelmed. Discussing your thoughts and worries with someone else might reduce stress and help you avoid emotional eating.

- Practice mindful eating: When you do eat, practice mindful eating by paying attention to your hunger and fullness cues. Eat slowly, savor each bite, and focus on the nourishment and enjoyment of the food.

Conclusion

This book is not just a book about shedding pounds; it is a guide to transforming your lifestyle and achieving sustainable weight loss. By implementing the strategies outlined in this book, such as creating healthy habits, building a support system, and managing stress and emotional eating, you will embark on a journey toward a version of yourself that is healthier, happier, and more self-assured.

The key to successful weight loss lies in making small, gradual changes that are manageable and sustainable. By focusing on balance in your diet, prioritizing physical activity, practicing mindful eating, and getting enough sleep, you will not only shed excess weight but also improve your overall well-being.

A strong support system is crucial on this journey. Whether it's enlisting the help of friends and family, joining a weight loss program or support group, or seeking professional guidance, having others by your side will provide encouragement, accountability, and motivation.

Another crucial component of long-term weight loss is controlling stress and emotional eating. By identifying triggers, finding alternative coping mechanisms, practicing self-care, and seeking support, you can overcome the obstacles that often derail progress and stay on track towards your goals.

Remember, this is not a one-size-fits-all approach. Each individual's journey is unique, and it's important to find the strategies that work best for you. With determination, perseverance, and the tools provided in this book, you have the power to achieve lasting weight loss and maintain your progress for a lifetime. So, take the first step towards a healthier future. Embrace the knowledge within these pages, implement the strategies outlined, and embark on a transformative journey towards a healthier, happier you. Your success awaits.